Introduction

Why Smart Weight Loss Matters
- Introduction to the concept of sustainable weight loss.
- The importance of a balanced approach to health and fitness.
- Overview of what readers can expect from the eBook.

Chapter 1: Understanding Weight Loss

The Science Behind Weight Loss
- How the body burns fat: metabolism, calories, and energy balance.
- The role of hormones in weight loss (insulin, cortisol, etc.).
- Myths vs. facts: Dispelling common misconceptions about dieting.

Setting Realistic Goals
- Understanding your body and setting achievable targets.
- The importance of tracking progress without obsessing over the scale.

Chapter 2: Nutrition - The Foundation of Smart Weight Loss

Eating for Weight Loss
- Calorie balance: How much to eat to lose weight.
- The importance of macronutrients (proteins, carbs, fats).
- Micronutrients and their role in metabolism and overall health.

Smart Food Choices
- The best foods for weight loss: whole foods, lean proteins, healthy fats.
- Foods to avoid: processed sugars, refined carbs, and empty calories.
- Portion control and mindful eating.

Meal Planning & Prep for Success
- Tips for creating a sustainable meal plan.
- Healthy snack ideas to keep cravings at bay.
- How to eat out and still stay on track with your goals.

Chapter 3: Exercise - Move to Lose

The Role of Exercise in Weight Loss
- Why exercise is key to both fat loss and muscle preservation.
- Cardiovascular exercise vs. strength training: Which is more effective?

- The importance of consistency over intensity.

Creating an Exercise Routine
- How to incorporate both cardio and strength training into your weekly schedule.
- The benefits of flexibility and mobility exercises (yoga, stretching).
- Effective home workouts for busy schedules.

Staying Motivated to Exercise
- Tips to make exercise a habit.
- Finding fun, enjoyable activities to stay active.
- Tracking progress and celebrating milestones.

Chapter 4: Lifestyle Habits That Support Weight Loss

Sleep and Weight Loss
- How inadequate sleep affects weight loss.
- Tips for improving sleep quality.
- The connection between stress, cortisol, and weight gain.

Managing Stress for Weight Loss
- Understanding stress and its impact on eating habits.
- Techniques for stress management: mindfulness, meditation, and relaxation practices.

Building Healthy Habits for Long-Term Success
- Developing a routine that supports weight loss goals.
- The role of consistency and small lifestyle changes.
- Overcoming obstacles and staying resilient.

Chapter 5: Common Pitfalls and How to Avoid Them

Dealing with Setbacks
- Understanding weight loss plateaus and how to break through them.
- How to stay positive and motivated when progress slows down.

Avoiding Fad Diets and Quick Fixes
- Why crash diets and extreme measures don't work long-term.
- How to identify and avoid weight loss scams.
- Sustainable, healthy approaches to permanent weight loss.

Overcoming Emotional Eating
- Recognizing triggers and patterns of emotional eating.
- Strategies to deal with stress, boredom, or emotional hunger without turning to food.

Chapter 6: Staying on Track - Long-Term Success

Maintaining Your New Lifestyle
- How to transition from weight loss mode to weight maintenance.
- Setting new health and fitness goals to keep the momentum going.
- Celebrating non-scale victories (improved energy, strength, confidence).

Building a Support System
- The importance of a support network: family, friends, or an accountability partner.
- Online communities and weight loss groups for motivation.
- Seeking professional help: nutritionists, trainers, and coaches.

Conclusion: Your Journey to a Healthier You

Recap of Key Tips for Smart Weight Loss
- Summarizing the most important takeaways from the eBook.
- Reinforcing the importance of patience, consistency, and self-compassion.

A Final Encouragement for the Road Ahead
- Empowering readers to embrace their weight loss journey.
- Encouraging ongoing growth and self-improvement.
- Invitation to continue learning, adapting, and thriving in their healthy lifestyle.

Bonus Section: Helpful Resources

Meal Plan Templates and Recipe Ideas
- Simple, nutritious recipes for weight loss.
- Easy-to-follow meal prep guides.

Workout Plans and Routines
- Example exercise routines for beginners, intermediate, and advanced levels.
- Tips for staying active throughout the day (e.g., walking, standing desks).

Recommended Apps & Tools for Tracking Progress
- Fitness trackers, meal logging apps, and weight loss trackers.

Frequently Asked Questions (FAQ)
- Answers to common weight loss questions.
- Troubleshooting tips for common challenges.

Introduction

Welcome to *"Shed Pounds the Smart Way: Top Weight Loss Tips You Need to Know."* If you've ever struggled with losing weight, or have tried various diets only to feel frustrated or discouraged, you're not alone. This eBook is designed to help you navigate the overwhelming world of weight loss with practical, science-backed strategies that promote long-term success. Here, we're focusing on sustainable weight loss—a gradual, healthy approach that ensures you don't just lose the pounds, but also keep them off for good.

In today's world, where diet fads and quick fixes often dominate, the importance of a **balanced approach to health and fitness** cannot be overstated. Losing weight isn't about drastic measures or shortcuts—it's about adopting healthy habits that you can maintain for the rest of your life. True transformation happens when we nourish our bodies with the right foods, incorporate exercise into our daily lives, and prioritize overall well-being, including sleep, stress management, and emotional health.

So, what can you expect from this eBook? In the following chapters, we'll break down weight loss into manageable steps that are not only effective but realistic. You'll learn about the science of weight loss, how to fuel your body with the right nutrients, the best ways to stay active, and strategies for managing your mental and emotional health along the way. We'll tackle common pitfalls, such as dealing with setbacks and overcoming emotional eating, and provide you with actionable tips to help you stay on track, even when the going gets tough.

This eBook is not just about shedding pounds; it's about building a healthier, more balanced lifestyle that will leave you feeling energized, confident, and proud of your progress. Let's get started on this exciting journey toward your best self!

Chapter 1: Understanding Weight Loss

Weight loss is a complex and often misunderstood process. Many people struggle with confusing information, misinformation, and contradictory advice. In this chapter, we'll break down the science of weight loss, highlight the role of hormones and metabolism, and help you set realistic, achievable goals for your journey. Understanding how weight loss works will give you the knowledge and confidence you need to make the right choices, avoid common mistakes, and stay on track to reach your health and fitness goals.

---

1. The Science Behind Weight Loss

At its core, weight loss is a simple concept: **calories in vs. calories out.** The energy your body uses comes from the calories you consume through food and beverages, and the energy it burns comes from basic metabolic processes and physical activity. If you consume more calories than your body burns, you gain weight. Conversely, if you consume fewer calories than you burn, your body starts using stored fat for energy, and you lose weight.

However, while the principle of calorie balance is fundamental, weight loss is more than just a numbers game. Your metabolism, hormones, and lifestyle habits play significant roles in how efficiently your body burns fat and maintains weight. Let's explore how these factors come into play.

---

2. How the Body Burns Fat: Metabolism, Calories, and Energy Balance

Metabolism is the process by which your body converts food into energy. It's the sum of all the chemical reactions in your body that keep you alive, from breathing to digesting food. Your metabolic rate, or the speed at which your body burns calories, varies from person to person and is influenced by several factors, including genetics, age, muscle mass, and activity levels.

There are three key components that determine how many calories your body burns:

- **Basal Metabolic Rate (BMR):** The number of calories your body needs to perform essential functions like breathing, circulation, and cell repair at rest. BMR accounts for the majority of the calories you burn each day.
- **Physical Activity:** This includes all forms of movement, from exercise to everyday activities like walking or cleaning. The more active you are, the more calories you burn.
- **Thermic Effect of Food (TEF):** The calories used to digest, absorb, and metabolize food. Certain foods, like protein, require more energy to process, which can slightly increase your calorie burn.

In simple terms, to lose weight, you need to create a calorie deficit, where the energy (calories) burned exceeds the energy consumed. This can be achieved by either eating fewer calories or increasing your physical activity—or ideally, a combination of both.

3. The Role of Hormones in Weight Loss

Hormones are chemical messengers in the body that regulate many physiological processes, including metabolism and appetite. Understanding how certain hormones impact weight loss can help you make smarter decisions on your journey. Here are a few key hormones involved in weight management:

- **Insulin:** Produced by the pancreas, insulin helps regulate blood sugar levels by facilitating the uptake of glucose (sugar) into cells for energy. High levels of insulin can promote fat storage, making it harder to lose weight. A diet high in processed carbs and sugars can lead to frequent insulin spikes, which can hinder weight loss efforts.
- **Cortisol:** Known as the "stress hormone," cortisol is released when you're stressed or in a fight-or-flight situation. While cortisol is necessary for survival, chronic stress and elevated cortisol levels can lead to increased fat storage, particularly around the abdomen. Managing stress is crucial for weight loss.
- **Leptin and Ghrelin:** Leptin is the "satiety hormone" that signals to your brain when you're full, while ghrelin is the "hunger hormone" that tells you when to eat. Poor sleep, stress, and dieting can disrupt the balance of these hormones, leading to increased hunger and cravings.

Balancing these hormones through a healthy diet, exercise, and stress management is essential for promoting fat loss and maintaining a healthy weight.

4. Myths vs. Facts: Dispelling Common Misconceptions About Dieting

When it comes to dieting and weight loss, there is no shortage of myths that can confuse and derail your progress. Here are a few of the most common misconceptions:

- **Myth: "Cutting carbs is the key to losing weight."**
  Fact: While reducing refined carbs (like white bread and sugary foods) can help with weight loss, carbs are an essential nutrient, and not all carbs are created equal. Whole grains, fruits, and vegetables are healthy sources of carbohydrates that can support weight loss and overall health.
- **Myth: "You have to exercise intensely to lose weight."**
  Fact: While intense workouts can be effective, consistency and the combination of both cardio and strength training are key. Exercise is important, but creating a calorie deficit through diet and long-term healthy habits is what truly drives weight loss.
- **Myth: "You have to be hungry to lose weight."**
  Fact: Sustainable weight loss is about fueling your body with the right foods in the right amounts, not starving yourself. A balanced, nutrient-dense diet will keep you satisfied while still enabling weight loss.
- **Myth: "Fad diets offer quick results."**
  Fact: Fad diets often lead to quick, unsustainable weight loss that is not maintained in the long term. They can also negatively affect your metabolism and overall health. The key is slow, steady progress with a focus on long-term habits.

5. Setting Realistic Goals

Setting goals is an essential part of any weight loss journey, but it's important to ensure those goals are realistic and achievable. Unrealistic expectations often lead to frustration and burnout. Here's how to approach goal-setting for lasting success:

6. Understanding Your Body and Setting Achievable Targets

Everyone's body is different, and what works for one person might not work for another. Understanding your body's unique needs and capabilities is crucial. Start by setting **small, specific goals** that align with your lifestyle and capabilities. These might include:

- Losing 1-2 pounds per week.
- Increasing your daily step count by 2,000 steps.
- Adding one additional workout per week.

These incremental goals help build momentum and are more sustainable over time than focusing on dramatic weight loss. Remember, weight loss is a marathon, not a sprint.

7. The Importance of Tracking Progress Without Obsessing Over the Scale

While tracking progress is important, it's essential to remember that the number on the scale is just one measure of success. **Non-scale victories** (NSVs) such as improved energy, better sleep, increased strength, or looser clothing can be just as meaningful—and sometimes more rewarding—than weight loss alone. Use the scale as a tool, but don't let it define your progress.

Tracking your food intake, workouts, sleep, and stress levels can provide a more comprehensive picture of your journey. Celebrate all the little victories, and understand that weight loss can fluctuate due to various factors like water retention or hormonal changes.

Chapter 2: Nutrition - The Foundation of Smart Weight Loss

When it comes to weight loss, nutrition is the foundation upon which all other aspects of your journey are built. While exercise is important, what you eat plays a more significant role in determining whether you lose weight and how quickly. The key to sustainable weight loss lies in making smart, nourishing food choices that fuel your body properly while creating a calorie deficit. In this chapter, we'll explore the essential elements of nutrition, including how to eat for weight loss, the importance of macronutrients and micronutrients, and how to make healthy food choices that support your goals.

---

1. Eating for Weight Loss

The concept of eating for weight loss begins with understanding how calories work. **Calories are the energy that our bodies derive from food.** If you consume more calories than your body needs, the excess will be stored as fat. Conversely, if you eat fewer calories than your body requires, your body will tap into stored fat for energy, leading to weight loss.

However, weight loss is not just about reducing calories—it's about ensuring the food you eat provides the nutrients your body needs to function at its best. Simply cutting calories without considering the nutritional value of your food can lead to deficiencies, low energy, and muscle loss, which can hinder your progress. Instead, aim to eat a variety of nutrient-dense foods that provide your body with what it needs to thrive, while also achieving a calorie deficit for fat loss.

---

2. Calorie Balance: How Much to Eat to Lose Weight

To lose weight, the most important factor is creating a **calorie deficit**. This means you must burn more calories than you consume. There are two main ways to achieve this: reduce your calorie intake or increase your physical activity. The general rule of thumb for safe and sustainable weight loss is to aim for a deficit of 500-1,000 calories per day, which typically results in losing 1-2 pounds per week.

To determine how much you should eat to lose weight, calculate your **Total Daily Energy Expenditure (TDEE)**, which takes into account your Basal Metabolic Rate (BMR) and your activity level. From there, subtract 500-1,000 calories to create your deficit. Many apps and websites can help you track your daily calorie intake, but it's also essential to listen to your body's hunger cues to avoid extreme calorie restriction.

---

3. The Importance of Macronutrients (Proteins, Carbs, Fats)

Macronutrients are the three main categories of nutrients that provide energy for the body. Understanding the role of each macronutrient will help you make the best choices for your weight loss goals.

- **Proteins**: Protein is essential for muscle repair and growth, and it plays a key role in satiety—helping you feel fuller for longer. Eating enough protein helps preserve lean muscle mass while losing fat. Aim to include a source of lean protein in every meal, such as chicken, fish, eggs, or plant-based options like beans and lentils.
- **Carbohydrates**: Carbs are your body's primary source of energy. However, not all carbs are equal. Choose complex carbs like whole grains, fruits, and vegetables, which are rich in fiber and nutrients. These foods help maintain steady energy levels and keep you satisfied longer. Avoid refined carbs, like white bread and pastries, which can cause blood sugar spikes and crashes.
- **Fats**: Healthy fats are essential for hormone production, brain function, and overall health. Include sources of unsaturated fats, such as avocados, nuts, seeds, and olive oil, in your diet. While fats are calorie-dense, they are also incredibly satiating and can help prevent overeating.

A balanced diet that includes all three macronutrients in appropriate proportions will keep your metabolism working efficiently and support fat loss without sacrificing muscle or energy.

---

4. Micronutrients and Their Role in Metabolism and Overall Health

While macronutrients are essential for providing energy, **micronutrients**—vitamins and minerals—are just as important for overall health and metabolic function. Micronutrients support processes like digestion, immune function, and energy production, which are crucial when you're losing weight.

For example, **vitamin D** helps with fat metabolism and immune function, while **magnesium** plays a role in regulating blood sugar. **B-vitamins** are important for energy production, and **iron** is necessary for oxygen transport in the blood. A nutrient-dense diet that includes a variety of colorful fruits, vegetables, whole grains, and lean proteins will ensure you're getting the micronutrients your body needs to function optimally during your weight loss journey.

---

5. Smart Food Choices

Making smart food choices is essential for both losing weight and maintaining overall health. While the number of calories you consume matters, it's also important to focus on the quality of those calories.

---

6. The Best Foods for Weight Loss: Whole Foods, Lean Proteins, Healthy Fats

Whole, minimally processed foods are the foundation of any smart weight loss plan. These foods are nutrient-dense, meaning they provide a lot of vitamins, minerals, and fiber without excess calories. Some examples of the best foods for weight loss include:

- **Lean proteins**: Chicken breast, turkey, fish, eggs, tofu, legumes, and low-fat dairy.

- **Vegetables**: Leafy greens, cruciferous vegetables (broccoli, cauliflower), carrots, peppers, zucchini, etc.
- **Fruits**: Berries, apples, oranges, bananas, and pears.
- **Whole grains**: Brown rice, quinoa, oats, barley, and whole wheat bread.
- **Healthy fats**: Olive oil, avocados, nuts, seeds, and fatty fish like salmon.

These foods are rich in fiber and protein, which help with satiety and provide essential nutrients without excess calories.

---

7. Foods to Avoid: Processed Sugars, Refined Carbs, and Empty Calories

To lose weight efficiently, it's important to minimize foods that provide little nutritional value, known as **empty calories**. These foods are typically high in refined sugars, unhealthy fats, and processed ingredients. Some foods to avoid include:

- **Sugary snacks**: Candy, cookies, cakes, and pastries.
- **Sugary beverages**: Sodas, sugary coffee drinks, and fruit juices.
- **Refined carbs**: White bread, white rice, and pasta made from refined flour.
- **Fried and processed foods**: Fast food, chips, and packaged snacks.

These foods can spike your blood sugar, cause insulin resistance, and lead to weight gain. Focus instead on whole, natural foods that nourish your body.

---

8. Portion Control and Mindful Eating

Even healthy foods can contribute to weight gain if consumed in large amounts. **Portion control** is key to losing weight without feeling deprived. Pay attention to serving sizes, and avoid eating large portions of calorie-dense foods like nuts, cheese, and oils.

Mindful eating is another powerful tool for weight loss. This involves paying full attention to your food—enjoying every bite, eating slowly, and tuning in to your hunger and fullness cues. By eating mindfully, you're less likely to overeat and more likely to enjoy your meals without guilt.

---

9. Meal Planning & Prep for Success

Successful weight loss requires organization and consistency. Planning ahead is one of the most effective ways to stay on track with your nutritional goals.

---

10. Tips for Creating a Sustainable Meal Plan

Creating a meal plan that suits your lifestyle is crucial for long-term success. Here are a few tips to get started:

- **Choose meals you enjoy**: If you hate eating salads, don't plan to eat them every day. Choose foods that satisfy you and fit into your calorie goals.
- **Batch cook and prep**: Prepare meals in advance to avoid the temptation of unhealthy options when you're hungry.
- **Include variety**: Eating the same meals every day can get boring, so mix it up with different proteins, vegetables, and grains.

---

11. Healthy Snack Ideas to Keep Cravings at Bay

Snacking doesn't have to sabotage your weight loss efforts. Healthy snacks can keep you full between meals and prevent overeating. Some great options include:

- Greek yogurt with berries
- Hummus and carrot sticks
- A handful of nuts or seeds
- A boiled egg and an apple
- Cottage cheese with cucumber slices

---

12. How to Eat Out and Still Stay on Track with Your Goals

Eating out doesn't have to mean derailing your progress. Here's how to stay on track when dining out:

- **Look for grilled or baked options** instead of fried.
- **Request dressings and sauces on the side** to control portion sizes.
- **Choose healthier sides** like steamed vegetables or a side salad.
- **Watch your portion sizes**—restaurant servings are often much larger than what you need.

With a little planning, you can enjoy dining out while still supporting your weight loss goals.

Chapter 3: Exercise - Move to Lose

Exercise is one of the most powerful tools for achieving and maintaining weight loss. While diet plays a major role in losing weight, **exercise is the engine that helps you burn fat, preserve muscle, and improve overall health.** Whether you're trying to shed pounds, build strength, or just feel better in your own skin, moving your body regularly is essential. In this chapter, we'll explore the role of exercise in weight loss, how to design an effective workout routine, and tips to keep you motivated throughout your fitness journey.

---

1. The Role of Exercise in Weight Loss

Exercise serves two critical functions in weight loss: **burning calories** and **preserving muscle mass**. When you create a calorie deficit through diet, your body will start to break down fat for energy. However, it can also break down muscle tissue, which is counterproductive if your goal is to lose fat and not lean mass. This is where exercise—especially strength training—becomes crucial.

When you exercise, especially with resistance or weight training, you signal your body to preserve and even build muscle while burning fat. This helps you keep your metabolism high, meaning you'll burn more calories even when you're not working out.

Moreover, cardiovascular exercise (like running or cycling) helps you burn calories and improves your cardiovascular health, contributing further to your calorie deficit and overall fat loss.

---

2. Why Exercise Is Key to Both Fat Loss and Muscle Preservation

Weight loss is not just about losing fat—it's about preserving lean muscle mass while shedding excess fat. **Muscle burns more calories at rest than fat**, which means having more muscle boosts your metabolism. Incorporating both cardio and strength training into your exercise routine ensures that you're burning fat, not muscle.

Strength training not only preserves muscle, but it also increases your strength and tone, contributing to a leaner, more sculpted body. It also has benefits for bone density, metabolism, and overall functional fitness. **Cardio, on the other hand, is excellent for fat loss**, improving heart health, and increasing endurance.

Combining both types of exercise in your weekly routine will provide a balanced approach to weight loss while maximizing results.

---

3. Cardiovascular Exercise vs. Strength Training: Which is More Effective?

Both cardiovascular exercise and strength training play vital roles in a balanced fitness plan, but each serves a different purpose when it comes to weight loss.

- **Cardiovascular Exercise**: Activities like walking, running, swimming, cycling, or dancing elevate your heart rate and burn calories quickly. While cardio is effective for burning fat during and after the workout, it doesn't do as much for preserving or building muscle. It's great for improving endurance and overall cardiovascular health, but it can lead to muscle loss if done excessively without strength training.
- **Strength Training**: Lifting weights or performing bodyweight exercises (like squats, lunges, and push-ups) is more about building lean muscle. Strength training helps to elevate your metabolism, build muscle mass, and reshape your body. It's essential for preserving muscle while losing fat and promoting long-term weight loss.

Which is more effective? The answer depends on your individual goals. For overall fat loss, a combination of both cardio and strength training is most effective. Aim for at least 2-3 strength training sessions per week, combined with 2-3 cardio sessions, for the best results.

---

4. The Importance of Consistency Over Intensity

One of the most important lessons in weight loss and fitness is that **consistency is far more important than intensity**. It's tempting to push yourself hard during every workout, but long-term results come from making exercise a consistent part of your lifestyle.

- **Intensity** can lead to burnout and injury if you try to go too hard, too fast. Short bursts of intense workouts can be effective but should be balanced with lower-intensity activities to ensure recovery.
- **Consistency**, on the other hand, ensures that you're regularly moving your body, improving endurance, building muscle, and burning calories over time. If you're consistent with your workouts, you'll see progress without the stress of trying to go all-out every session.

Focus on **creating a regular exercise schedule** and gradually increase intensity as your body adapts. It's better to commit to 30 minutes of moderate exercise, five times a week, than to do a few intense sessions that leave you feeling drained or injured.

---

5. Creating an Exercise Routine

When it comes to weight loss, the key to success lies in a well-rounded fitness routine that combines cardio, strength training, and flexibility exercises. But how do you create a plan that works for you? Here's how:

---

6. How to Incorporate Both Cardio and Strength Training Into Your Weekly Schedule

To lose weight effectively, aim to **incorporate both cardio and strength training into your weekly routine**. Here's a simple framework to help you get started:

- **Strength Training**: Aim for 2-3 strength training sessions per week. These can be full-body workouts or split routines (focusing on different muscle groups each session).
- **Cardio**: Include 2-3 cardio sessions per week. You can choose from low-impact exercises like walking, or more intense activities like running or cycling.
- **Rest and Recovery**: Incorporate at least one or two rest days per week to allow your muscles to recover and rebuild.

Here's an example of a weekly schedule:

- **Monday**: Full-body strength training
- **Tuesday**: Cardio (e.g., 30-minute brisk walk or jog)
- **Wednesday**: Upper body strength training
- **Thursday**: Cardio (e.g., cycling or swimming)
- **Friday**: Lower body strength training
- **Saturday**: Active rest (e.g., yoga, stretching, or a light walk)
- **Sunday**: Rest day

This schedule provides a balance of strength training and cardio while giving your body the recovery time it needs.

---

7. The Benefits of Flexibility and Mobility Exercises (Yoga, Stretching)

While cardio and strength training are essential for weight loss, **flexibility and mobility exercises** should not be overlooked. These exercises help improve the range of motion in your joints, increase blood flow, and prevent injury.

Yoga and stretching can enhance your overall fitness routine by promoting muscle recovery, reducing muscle tightness, and improving posture. Including regular stretching or yoga sessions in your routine will also help relieve stress and keep you motivated by improving how your body feels.

Incorporate at least one or two sessions of yoga or stretching into your weekly plan for a balanced approach to fitness.

---

8. Effective Home Workouts for Busy Schedules

Not everyone has the time or resources to go to the gym. The good news is that you can achieve significant weight loss results from the comfort of your own home with effective home workouts. Here are a few ideas:

- **Bodyweight exercises**: Push-ups, squats, lunges, and planks are all excellent for strength training at home.
- **HIIT (High-Intensity Interval Training)**: These short bursts of intense exercise followed by rest periods can torch calories and improve endurance in a short amount of time.
- **Jump rope**: A fantastic cardio option that takes up minimal space and can be done anywhere.
- **Online workout classes**: There are plenty of free or subscription-based workout programs that cater to all levels and allow you to work out at home.

With minimal equipment or no equipment at all, you can still achieve an effective workout at home.

---

9. Staying Motivated to Exercise

Staying motivated can be one of the hardest parts of any fitness journey. Here are some strategies to help you stay committed:

---

10. Tips to Make Exercise a Habit

- **Start small**: Don't overwhelm yourself by trying to do too much at once. Start with short, manageable workouts and gradually build up.
- **Schedule workouts**: Treat your exercise routine like an important appointment that you can't skip.
- **Find accountability**: Partner with a friend, join a fitness class, or use a fitness app to track your progress.

---

11. Finding Fun, Enjoyable Activities to Stay Active

Exercise doesn't have to feel like a chore. Find activities that you enjoy, whether it's dancing, hiking, playing a sport, or doing yoga. When you enjoy your workouts, you're more likely to stick with them. Try different things until you find what works for you.

---

12. Tracking Progress and Celebrating Milestones

Tracking your progress—whether through a fitness app, journaling, or photos—can help keep you motivated and give you a sense of accomplishment. It's important to **celebrate milestones** along the way, whether it's a new personal best in your workouts, improved endurance, or feeling more energized.

Focus not just on the number on the scale, but on other positive changes like increased strength, better sleep, or improved mood.

Chapter 4: Lifestyle Habits That Support Weight Loss

When it comes to losing weight, **exercise** and **nutrition** often take center stage, but **lifestyle habits** can play a massive role in determining your success. **Sleep, stress management, and consistent healthy habits** are often overlooked but are essential for creating a foundation for lasting weight loss. In this chapter, we will explore how sleep affects weight loss, the role of stress in your weight loss journey, and the importance of building healthy habits to ensure long-term success.

---

1. Sleep and Weight Loss

Good sleep is not just about feeling rested—**it's a crucial factor in weight management**. When you don't get enough sleep, your body's hormones become imbalanced, which can make weight loss more difficult. Lack of sleep can lead to increased hunger, cravings for unhealthy foods, and a slower metabolism.

---

2. How Inadequate Sleep Affects Weight Loss

Inadequate sleep affects two primary hormones related to hunger: **ghrelin** and **leptin**.

- **Ghrelin**, the hunger hormone, increases when you're sleep-deprived, making you feel hungrier and more likely to crave high-calorie foods.
- **Leptin**, the hormone that signals fullness, decreases with poor sleep, so even when you eat, you may still feel hungry.

Additionally, chronic sleep deprivation can impair your metabolism and the body's ability to process food effectively, which may lead to weight gain over time. **Sleep also impacts insulin sensitivity**, which affects how your body stores and processes fat. If you're not getting quality rest, your body may be more prone to storing excess calories as fat.

---

3. Tips for Improving Sleep Quality

To optimize your sleep and make it a supportive factor in your weight loss journey, try the following tips:

- **Create a bedtime routine**: A consistent pre-sleep routine can signal your body that it's time to wind down. Try reading, stretching, or practicing relaxation techniques before bed.
- **Avoid screen time before bed**: The blue light emitted by phones, computers, and TVs can interfere with your body's ability to produce melatonin, the hormone that helps you sleep.
- **Make your sleep environment comfortable**: Ensure your room is cool, dark, and quiet. Consider using blackout curtains, earplugs, or a white noise machine if needed.
- **Limit caffeine and alcohol**: These substances can disrupt your sleep cycle, so avoid them, especially in the afternoon and evening.
- **Aim for 7-9 hours of sleep per night**: Consistent, high-quality sleep is key to regulating hormones and supporting weight loss efforts.

---

4. The Connection Between Stress, Cortisol, and Weight Gain

Stress can wreak havoc on your body in many ways, and one of the most significant impacts is on your weight. When you experience stress, your body releases a hormone called **cortisol**. Cortisol is often referred to as the "stress hormone" because it helps you respond to stressful situations by triggering the "fight or flight" response. However, chronic stress and prolonged elevated cortisol levels can contribute to **weight gain**, particularly around the abdomen.

High cortisol levels lead to **increased appetite**, especially for high-fat, sugary foods. This creates a cycle where stress leads to overeating, and overeating leads to weight gain, which in turn increases stress. It can also affect your metabolism, making it harder for your body to burn fat effectively.

---

5. Managing Stress for Weight Loss

Managing stress is a crucial step in your weight loss journey. Finding ways to cope with stress can help you prevent emotional eating and curb cravings, making it easier to stick to your weight loss goals.

---

6. Understanding Stress and Its Impact on Eating Habits

When we're stressed, we're more likely to make poor food choices—often seeking comfort in **processed foods**, **sugary snacks**, or **high-fat comfort foods**. This type of eating is sometimes referred to as **emotional eating**. It's important to recognize when stress is influencing your eating habits and take steps to address the root cause of the stress rather than using food as a coping mechanism.

Stress can also lead to **increased food consumption** in some individuals, while others may lose their appetite entirely. This variance in stress response can make it challenging to find balance and consistency in your eating habits.

---

7. Techniques for Stress Management: Mindfulness, Meditation, and Relaxation Practices

To manage stress effectively, it's important to build healthy coping strategies. Consider incorporating these practices into your routine:

- **Mindfulness and Meditation**: Mindfulness involves paying attention to the present moment without judgment. It can help reduce stress by allowing you to become aware of your thoughts and emotions, helping you avoid reacting impulsively, especially with food. Meditation can lower cortisol levels and promote relaxation, making it easier to manage stress and cravings.
- **Breathing Exercises**: Deep breathing exercises, such as diaphragmatic breathing, can help activate the parasympathetic nervous system, which helps calm the body and reduce stress. Take a few minutes each day to practice deep breathing when you feel stressed.
- **Progressive Muscle Relaxation**: This technique involves tensing and then relaxing different muscle groups to relieve physical tension and reduce stress. It's especially helpful if you carry stress in your body, such as in your shoulders or back.
- **Physical Activity**: Exercise is one of the most effective stress relievers. Whether it's a walk, yoga, or a full workout, physical activity helps release endorphins, which are the body's natural mood elevators.

---

8. Building Healthy Habits for Long-Term Success

Sustainable weight loss is not a quick fix—it requires consistent habits that support your overall well-being. Establishing a routine and sticking to it is critical for long-term success. Here's how you can build healthy habits that work for you.

---

9. Developing a Routine That Supports Weight Loss Goals

A solid routine can provide structure and consistency to your weight loss efforts. When you establish healthy habits, such as meal prepping, exercising regularly, and getting enough sleep, it becomes easier to stay on track.

- **Plan your meals and workouts**: Block off time for both meal prep and exercise each week. Creating a consistent schedule will help you stay committed and prevent you from falling off track due to time constraints.

- **Start your day with a positive morning routine**: A productive morning sets the tone for the rest of the day. Incorporate habits such as hydration, stretching, and a healthy breakfast to set you up for success.

---

10. The Role of Consistency and Small Lifestyle Changes

Weight loss isn't about perfection—it's about **consistency**. Small, incremental changes in your lifestyle are more sustainable than drastic changes that can be hard to maintain. Focus on making small adjustments, such as cutting back on sugary drinks, increasing your daily steps, or swapping out processed snacks for healthier options. These minor changes add up over time and lead to significant, lasting results.

---

11. Overcoming Obstacles and Staying Resilient

Throughout your weight loss journey, you will encounter challenges. Whether it's a weight loss plateau, a busy schedule, or moments of self-doubt, it's essential to stay resilient. Here's how you can overcome obstacles:

- **Stay patient**: Weight loss takes time. Focus on the small victories, such as increased energy, better sleep, and improved fitness.
- **Don't be too hard on yourself**: Slip-ups are part of the process. If you have a setback, don't give up. Get back on track the next day, and remember that progress is a journey.
- **Seek support**: Whether it's a workout buddy, a support group, or a coach, having people to encourage and motivate you can make a big difference in staying on track.

Chapter 5: Common Pitfalls and How to Avoid Them

Embarking on a weight loss journey is exciting, but it's also filled with challenges. Understanding and navigating common pitfalls can make the difference between success and frustration. In this chapter, we will explore how to handle setbacks, avoid quick-fix diets, and overcome emotional eating. By recognizing and addressing these obstacles, you'll be better equipped to stay on track and achieve sustainable, long-term weight loss.

---

1. Dealing with Setbacks

Weight loss isn't always a linear process. It's common to face setbacks along the way, whether it's a bad week of eating, a missed workout, or a sudden weight gain. The key to success lies not in avoiding setbacks, but in **how you respond to them**.

Setbacks can feel discouraging, but they don't define your progress. Rather than giving up, use setbacks as learning opportunities. Reflect on what happened, identify any triggers or challenges, and plan ways to handle them better in the future. **A positive mindset is crucial**—remember, weight loss is a marathon, not a sprint.

---

2. Understanding Weight Loss Plateaus and How to Break Through Them

At some point during your weight loss journey, you may encounter a plateau—a period where your progress seems to stall. This is frustrating, but it's a natural part of the process. Your body is simply adjusting to the changes, and you may need to make some modifications to keep moving forward.

Plateaus occur when your body adapts to your routine, reducing its energy expenditure. To break through a plateau:

- **Adjust your calorie intake**: If you've been on a calorie deficit for a while, your body may have adapted. Try lowering your calorie intake slightly or increasing your activity level.
- **Change up your workouts**: The body becomes accustomed to the same exercises over time. Try adding new activities or increasing the intensity of your workouts.
- **Prioritize sleep and stress management**: Both sleep and stress can contribute to plateaus. Make sure you're getting enough rest and keeping your cortisol levels under control.

Above all, **be patient**. Plateaus are temporary, and with the right adjustments, you will continue to make progress.

---

3. How to Stay Positive and Motivated When Progress Slows Down

When progress slows, it's easy to feel discouraged. However, it's important to remind yourself that **weight loss is a journey**—not every day will feel like a victory, but consistency over time leads to success.

- **Celebrate non-scale victories**: Weight isn't the only measure of success. Celebrate improvements in energy, strength, fitness, or even how your clothes fit. These victories are just as important as the number on the scale.
- **Focus on the process, not just the outcome**: Shift your mindset from focusing solely on the end goal to enjoying the journey. Appreciate how exercise makes you feel, how nourishing foods support your body, and how your lifestyle is transforming.

- **Stay connected to your "why"**: Remind yourself why you started this journey in the first place. Whether it's improving your health, feeling more confident, or being able to keep up with your kids, reconnecting with your reasons can help reignite your motivation.

---

4. Avoiding Fad Diets and Quick Fixes

It's tempting to chase quick results with fad diets or extreme weight loss measures. However, **short-term solutions** often lead to long-term frustration. These quick fixes may help you lose weight initially, but they are unsustainable and can have negative effects on your metabolism, health, and mental well-being.

---

5. Why Crash Diets and Extreme Measures Don't Work Long-Term

Crash diets often promise dramatic weight loss in a short period, but they come with a range of problems:

- **Nutrient deficiencies**: Many extreme diets cut out important food groups, leading to deficiencies that can harm your body over time.
- **Slower metabolism**: Extreme calorie restriction can slow down your metabolism, making it harder to lose weight in the future.
- **Muscle loss**: Severe dieting can lead to the loss of lean muscle mass, which is crucial for maintaining a healthy metabolism.

The biggest issue with crash diets is that they're unsustainable. Once you return to your normal eating habits, the weight often comes back—sometimes with a few extra pounds.

---

6. How to Identify and Avoid Weight Loss Scams

The weight loss industry is flooded with products and programs promising miracle results. Unfortunately, many of these are **scams** or short-lived fixes. Here's how to spot them:

- **Too good to be true**: If a product promises extreme results with little effort or time, it's likely a scam.
- **Lack of evidence**: Avoid programs that don't offer credible scientific evidence or professional endorsements. Look for information from reputable sources.
- **Quick-fix solutions**: Be wary of pills, supplements, or special foods that promise rapid weight loss. Sustainable weight loss requires lifestyle changes, not magic pills.

Stick to evidence-based methods that prioritize **healthy eating, regular exercise, and consistent habits**. Avoid falling for promises that sound too good to be true.

---

7. Sustainable, Healthy Approaches to Permanent Weight Loss

Instead of relying on quick fixes, focus on **long-term strategies** for weight loss that emphasize gradual, sustainable changes:

- **Balanced nutrition**: Eat whole, nutrient-dense foods that nourish your body. Avoid extremes and focus on moderation.
- **Regular exercise**: Incorporate both cardio and strength training to improve fat loss and preserve muscle mass.
- **Lifestyle changes**: Develop habits that support a healthy, active lifestyle. Create routines that incorporate sleep, stress management, and mindful eating.

By focusing on sustainable changes rather than drastic measures, you're more likely to see lasting results and avoid the frustration of regaining lost weight.

---

8. Overcoming Emotional Eating

Emotional eating is a common challenge for many people. When emotions like stress, sadness, or boredom arise, food can become a coping mechanism. **Emotional eating** can derail your weight loss efforts and lead to unhealthy eating habits.

---

9. Recognizing Triggers and Patterns of Emotional Eating

To overcome emotional eating, the first step is **awareness**. Start by identifying the triggers that lead to emotional eating:

- **Stress**: You may turn to food to soothe feelings of anxiety or pressure.
- **Boredom**: Eating out of boredom can be a way to pass the time, not because you're physically hungry.
- **Sadness or loneliness**: Food can sometimes provide comfort when you're feeling down.

Once you identify your emotional eating patterns, you can begin to find healthier ways to cope with your emotions, rather than using food as an emotional crutch.

---

10. Strategies to Deal with Stress, Boredom, or Emotional Hunger Without Turning to Food

Here are some effective strategies to manage emotional eating:

- **Pause and assess**: When you feel the urge to eat emotionally, pause and ask yourself if you're truly hungry or if you're trying to satisfy an emotional need. If you're not hungry, try to distract yourself with a different activity.

- **Find healthier coping mechanisms**: Engage in activities that soothe you without involving food—take a walk, practice deep breathing, meditate, or talk to a friend.
- **Stay hydrated**: Sometimes thirst is mistaken for hunger. Make sure you're drinking enough water throughout the day.
- **Practice mindful eating**: Be present when you eat. Focus on the taste, texture, and enjoyment of your food. This helps prevent mindless eating when emotions are running high.

By developing healthier coping mechanisms and becoming more mindful of emotional eating triggers, you can regain control over your eating habits and continue progressing toward your goals.

Chapter 6: Staying on Track - Long-Term Success

Achieving weight loss is a remarkable accomplishment, but the real challenge begins when it's time to **maintain** your progress over the long term. This chapter will guide you through the process of maintaining your new lifestyle, setting fresh goals, celebrating non-scale victories, and building a solid support system to help keep you on track for lasting success.

---

1. Maintaining Your New Lifestyle

After achieving your weight loss goals, it's essential to focus on maintaining the new habits and lifestyle that got you there. This transition can feel daunting, but with the right mindset and strategies, you can make it smooth and sustainable.

One of the biggest challenges people face after reaching their goal weight is **avoiding the temptation to return to old habits**. It's important to view this phase not as a "maintenance mode," but as a **lifestyle** that you'll continue to build on. Your focus should shift from restriction and weight loss to health and well-being. Keep making **mindful choices** that prioritize nutrition, regular exercise, and self-care, just as you did during your weight loss phase.

- **Make adjustments**: As your body adapts, your calorie needs may change. Reassess your caloric intake and exercise routine periodically to avoid weight regain.
- **Stay flexible**: Life happens, and some days may not go according to plan. The key is to remain flexible and get back on track without guilt or shame.

---

2. How to Transition from Weight Loss Mode to Weight Maintenance

The transition from weight loss mode to weight maintenance requires a shift in mindset. During weight loss, you were focused on **creating a calorie deficit**, but during maintenance, the goal is to **stabilize** and find balance.

Here's how to make the transition:

- **Gradually increase calories**: Slowly add more calories back into your diet to find your maintenance level without gaining back unwanted weight. This should be done in small increments to avoid overwhelming your metabolism.
- **Shift focus to performance**: Rather than obsessing over the scale, focus on **improving your fitness and strength**. Aim to enhance your endurance, flexibility, or strength with each workout.

- **Practice mindful eating**: Pay attention to your hunger and fullness cues, and avoid eating out of habit or boredom. This helps prevent overeating and promotes a healthy relationship with food.

---

3. Setting New Health and Fitness Goals to Keep the Momentum Going

Just because you've reached your weight loss goals doesn't mean you stop setting new ones. In fact, **setting new health and fitness goals** is crucial for maintaining your success and staying motivated. Here's how to keep the momentum going:

- **Set performance-based goals**: Instead of focusing solely on the number on the scale, set goals related to fitness, strength, or endurance. For example, challenge yourself to run a 5K, increase the amount of weight you can lift, or master a yoga pose.
- **Continue to track progress**: While weight may not be the focus anymore, keep track of other progress indicators, such as how your clothes fit, your energy levels, or improvements in physical performance.
- **Mix things up**: Try new activities or workouts to keep things interesting. Whether it's a new sport, fitness class, or outdoor activity, variety will keep you engaged and prevent boredom.

By setting new challenges, you'll continue to evolve and push yourself towards further improvement.

---

4. Celebrating Non-Scale Victories (Improved Energy, Strength, Confidence)

It's easy to get fixated on the scale, but **non-scale victories** are often much more important in the long run. These victories are the real markers of success and lasting change. Celebrating these achievements helps reinforce your motivation and gives you a deeper sense of fulfillment.

- **Improved energy**: One of the first things people notice when they lose weight and adopt a healthier lifestyle is a **boost in energy**. If you're sleeping better, eating nutritious foods, and exercising regularly, your overall energy levels will improve.
- **Strength and fitness**: Whether it's lifting heavier weights, running faster, or achieving a personal best in a workout, **physical strength** is a significant achievement.
- **Increased confidence**: As you maintain your weight loss and continue to improve your health, you'll likely notice an **increase in confidence** and self-esteem. Whether it's feeling more comfortable in your body or receiving compliments from others, confidence is a vital non-scale victory.
- **Improved health markers**: Many people experience positive changes in **blood pressure**, **cholesterol levels**, or **blood sugar** after losing weight and adopting a healthier lifestyle. These improvements are signs that your body is benefiting from your efforts beyond just your appearance.

Celebrating these milestones is essential for staying positive and maintaining momentum.

5. Building a Support System

A strong support system is one of the most important factors in maintaining long-term success. Surrounding yourself with people who encourage you and hold you accountable can make a huge difference in your weight loss and maintenance journey.

6. The Importance of a Support Network: Family, Friends, or an Accountability Partner

Having a **support network** can provide both emotional and practical support as you work toward your goals. Whether it's family, friends, or a **dedicated accountability partner**, knowing that someone is cheering you on and holding you accountable can motivate you to keep going.

- **Family and friends**: Share your journey with loved ones who support your healthy lifestyle. They can help you stay on track by offering encouragement, joining you for workouts, or providing healthy meal options.
- **Accountability partners**: Whether it's a friend, coworker, or online support group, an accountability partner can be a powerful motivator. Regularly check in with each other to track progress, discuss challenges, and celebrate successes.

7. Online Communities and Weight Loss Groups for Motivation

In addition to your personal support network, **online communities and weight loss groups** can offer additional motivation and connection. These groups can provide a sense of belonging and a platform for sharing experiences and challenges.

- **Find groups that align with your values**: There are countless online groups dedicated to healthy living, fitness, and weight loss. Find one that resonates with your goals and values.
- **Join in discussions**: Participate in conversations, share your progress, and ask for advice. These groups are a great place to exchange tips and experiences and feel supported along the way.

Online communities provide a broader support system and help you stay motivated even on tough days.

8. Seeking Professional Help: Nutritionists, Trainers, and Coaches

Sometimes, professional guidance can help you maintain your progress and fine-tune your routine. Seeking help from professionals like **nutritionists, personal trainers, or health coaches** can ensure that you stay on track and make any necessary adjustments to your plan.

- **Nutritionists** can help you develop a sustainable eating plan tailored to your needs and preferences.
- **Personal trainers** can provide workout plans that fit your fitness level and goals while ensuring you stay safe and effective in your routines.
- **Health coaches** can support you with goal-setting, motivation, and accountability to help you stay focused on your long-term success.

Hiring a professional might be an investment, but it can pay off in helping you maintain your progress and continue to thrive.

Conclusion: Your Journey to a Healthier, Happier You

As we reach the end of this eBook, it's important to take a step back and reflect on the key principles that have guided you throughout your weight loss journey. This is just the beginning of a new chapter in your life—one focused on **sustainable health**, **well-being**, and **personal growth**. Let's recap the most important tips and takeaways that will empower you to continue on your path with confidence and success.

---

1. Recap of Key Tips for Smart Weight Loss

- **Understanding weight loss**: It's not about drastic diets or extreme measures, but about creating a **caloric deficit** through balanced eating, exercise, and lifestyle changes. Your body burns fat when you manage your energy balance effectively, and by understanding the role of hormones like insulin and cortisol, you can better support your weight loss efforts.
- **Nutrition**: The foundation of any successful weight loss journey lies in **eating a balanced diet**. Prioritize whole, nutrient-dense foods such as lean proteins, healthy fats, and complex carbohydrates. Portion control and mindful eating are essential for avoiding overconsumption, and **meal planning** can make healthy eating both easy and sustainable.
- **Exercise**: Incorporating both **cardiovascular exercise** and **strength training** into your routine is key to burning fat and preserving muscle. Consistency is more important than intensity, and finding enjoyable activities will help you stick to an exercise routine over the long term. Flexibility and mobility exercises are also important for overall health.
- **Lifestyle habits**: Quality **sleep** and **stress management** are just as important as exercise and nutrition. Prioritize sleep, manage stress with mindfulness and relaxation techniques, and build **healthy habits** that support your weight loss goals. These habits should evolve into a long-term, sustainable routine.
- **Avoiding pitfalls**: Be cautious of **fad diets** and **quick fixes**—they may offer short-term results, but they are unsustainable in the long run. Focus on **building healthy habits** that will keep you on track for lasting success. Don't forget to address **emotional eating**, and recognize triggers so that you can approach food mindfully.

---

2. Reinforcing the Importance of Patience, Consistency, and Self-Compassion

As you continue your journey, it's essential to remember that **patience** is key. **Weight loss** is not a race—it's a gradual process that requires consistency over time. You will face setbacks and obstacles, but remember, these are part of the journey. Embrace the process, be patient with yourself, and always give yourself grace.

Consistency is what turns new habits into lasting change. Whether it's maintaining a healthy diet, sticking with a workout routine, or getting adequate rest, small, consistent efforts yield the best results.

Above all, practice **self-compassion**. Celebrate your progress, no matter how small, and don't beat yourself up over occasional slip-ups. You are learning, growing, and improving with every step.

---

3. A Final Encouragement for the Road Ahead

This is your journey. It's not about perfection—it's about progress. As you move forward, remember that your weight loss goals are not just about how you look on the outside, but how you feel on the inside. **Embrace the changes you are making**, and be proud of the effort you are putting in.

The key to lasting success is an **ongoing commitment** to self-improvement and personal growth. Stay open to new experiences, new knowledge, and new ways to support your health.

You will encounter challenges, but always remember: setbacks are temporary. What matters most is your **resilience** and your ability to **adapt**. With the right mindset, dedication, and tools, you can thrive in your healthy lifestyle.

---

4. Bonus Section: Helpful Resources

To support you on your journey, I've compiled a list of valuable **resources** to help you continue learning and thriving in your weight loss and fitness journey.

Meal Plan Templates and Recipe Ideas

Simple, Nutritious Recipes for Weight Loss
Here are some easy-to-follow recipes to kickstart your healthy eating. From breakfast options like protein-packed smoothies to dinner ideas like grilled chicken salads, these meals are designed to keep you full and satisfied while supporting your weight loss goals.

Easy-to-Follow Meal Prep Guides
Meal prepping is a great way to stay on track with healthy eating, even during busy weeks. Get tips and strategies for meal prepping in advance, along with a list of make-ahead recipes that keep your meals both delicious and nutritious.

Workout Plans and Routines

Exercise Routines for Beginners, Intermediate, and Advanced Levels
Whether you're just starting out or looking for more advanced workouts, you'll find routine examples that fit your fitness level. From beginner-friendly bodyweight exercises to advanced strength training and cardio, these routines will keep you motivated and moving toward your goals.

Tips for Staying Active Throughout the Day
Incorporating movement into your day doesn't have to be limited to your workout. Small changes—like walking more, using standing desks, or taking the stairs—can help you stay active and burn extra calories throughout the day.

Recommended Apps & Tools for Tracking Progress

Use technology to your advantage by tracking your progress and staying motivated:

- **Fitness Trackers**: Apps that track your steps, calories burned, and workouts.
- **Meal Logging Apps**: Tools to help you stay on top of your calorie intake and nutrition.
- **Weight Loss Trackers**: Use apps that help monitor your weight, measurements, and other health markers to ensure you're on track.

Frequently Asked Questions (FAQ)

In this section, you'll find answers to some of the most commonly asked questions about weight loss, including how to break through plateaus, stay motivated when progress slows down, and manage emotional eating. We've also included some troubleshooting tips for common challenges.

Your Journey is Just Beginning

The journey to health and wellness is lifelong. With the tools, tips, and resources shared in this book, you have everything you need to **succeed**—but the most important ingredient is **you**. Keep pushing forward, stay committed to your goals, and most importantly, **enjoy the journey**. You've got this!

Stay healthy, stay strong, and keep thriving.